TABLE OF CONTENTS

HIDDEN STRESS AND ILLNESS IN WOMEN

10 SYMPTOMS OF HIDDEN STRESS IN WOMEN

1 VASOVAGAL

2. DECREASED IMMUNE SYSTEM

3. POOR DIGESTION

4. ACNE

5. HEADACHES

6. POOR DIET

7. LIBIDO DECREASE

8. APPETITE CHANGES

9. MUSCLE TENSION

10. RAPID HEART BEAT

PHYSICAL CONSEQUENCES OF HIDDEN STRESS IN WOMEN

Brain and ears

Cardiovascular System

Upset stomach

Diabetes

Tense muscles

Increased skin disease

PSYCHOLOGICAL CONSEQUENCES OF STRESS

Fear and anger

HIDDEN STRESS AND ILLNESS IN WOMEN

Stress is a state of mind and body that is triggered by undesirable conditions. Each person's body portrays stress symptoms in different ways, from external symptoms such as facial acne to internal symptoms such as chronic diseases. When stress is not controlled, it can cause many signs and symptoms.

Stress is our physical performance when we feel overwhelmed and unable to cope with the needs of life. These needs may be related to anything from work, school, family, or friends. People of all ages may also cause stress because stress depends not only on the severity of the situation but also on people's ability to live and cope at the time.

Stress can also be used as a driving force and is an essential part of survival. The "fight or escape" mechanism can tell us how and when to deal with danger, which is a life-saving instinct. Unfortunately, when chronic stress triggers this mechanism too much, it may affect a person's physical and mental health.

10 SYMPTOMS OF HIDDEN STRESS IN WOMEN

1 VASOVAGAL

This stress symptom occurs when your body overreacts to triggers (such as emotional distress). It causes a sudden drop in your heart rate and blood pressure and reduces blood flow to the brain. This leads to loss of consciousness and syncope. The vagus nerve is usually harmless and does not require treatment, but syncope is very dangerous because you may be injured.

Before fainting from vagal vertigo, a person may experience the following symptoms: pale skin, dizziness, nausea, yawning, blurred vision, and sweating. Recovery usually starts quickly, but if you stand too early, there is a risk of syncope again.

Women may not always have the ability to avoid vasovagal nerves, and some women are more inclined to vasovagal nerves than others, but if you feel you may faint, lie down and raise your legs to keep gravity flowing to the brain.

2. DECREASED IMMUNE SYSTEM

The main type of immune cells is white blood cells, also called lymphocytes. When a woman is under stress, their cortisol levels increase, suppressing the effectiveness of the immune system and reducing the number of lymphocytes in the body. This will inhibit the body's ability to resist antigens, making us more susceptible to infection.

Stress can also indirectly affect the immune system. When women are under stress, they are more likely to eat unhealthy food, cigarettes or drinks. These behavioral coping strategies can temporarily relieve stress symptoms, but may also eventually trigger an immune response.

3. POOR DIGESTION

During stress, digestion is reserved, and after stress, digestion is increased. Studies have shown that epinephrine released during the stress response may be directly related to the development of ulcers.

Helicobacter pylori are the cause of some gastric ulcers. It lives in your digestive tract and can cause sores. Studies have shown that psychological stress can enhance the colonization of Helicobacter pylori in the stomach.

4. ACNE

Acne is one of the most obvious ways in which stress can manifest. The release of cortisol into the blood affects hormonal balance, which in turn leads to acne. Stressful women also tend to touch their faces and spread bacteria, thus promoting acne development.

The increase in acne may be caused due to increased endothelial secretion during periods of stress. Another theory is that the body responds to stress by directing blood flow and oxygen to areas that fight stress and withdrawing it from areas such as the skin. Insufficient blood and oxygen in the skin lead to clogged pores and broken pores. One study even suggested that women with acne experience more severe symptoms during exams and stressful periods. This suggests that emotional stress may have an important effect on acne. If you have stress-related acne, consider using quick-acting spot treatment or products that are used with salicylic acid, probiotics, or benzoyl peroxide to kill bacteria and reduce redness and inflammation. Be sure to exfoliate to remove dead cells and help clog pores. Exfoliation is the most beneficial way to remove dead skin cells and eliminate skin congestion. You should always consult an expert for diagnosis and appropriate treatment options.

5. HEADACHES

Many studies have also shown that stress may cause stiff neck muscles and cause headaches. It is one of the most common causes of tension-related headaches and may even cause migraines. Simple steps like meditation can help prevent stress from interfering with daily activities.

Daily stressors, such as women in work, traffic, or email, usually cope by grinding their teeth or tightening their necks. It's best to identify when this happens and take some time to organize and make yourself feel more in control of the stressor. Studies have shown that experiencing a large number of stressful events can also lead to insomnia.

Lack of sleep is a typical result of stress and can exacerbate women who are prone to headaches. Try to set the sleep time every night to 7 to 8 hours, and follow the regular sleep schedule. Try to lie in bed at the same time every night and wake up at the same time every morning. Changing your sleep style will negatively affect your sleep ability and may exacerbate stress-related insomnia.

6. POOR DIET

Under stress will inevitably lead to wrong decisions about diet. Following a diet rich in complex carbohydrates and healthy fats can help improve headaches and give women more control over the stress they are under. A balanced diet can affect the duration and intensity of headaches.
The vital tip is to maintain a healthy and balanced diet throughout the day. Start with a protein-containing breakfast, such as high-protein cereals or eggs. Eat brunch before lunch, so you don't feel tired and easily make bad food choices. Eat a balanced lunch, then snacks, and then dinner, always making sure you are not hungry or starved to death during the day. In this way, when the night comes, your blood sugar will be balanced, and you will feel satisfied and full.

7. LIBIDO DECREASE

It is not uncommon for sexual desire to decrease during times of tension. When your body reacts to stress, you will go through a series of changes to prepare to escape, which is a "fight or escape" response. This can be attributed to cortisol or epinephrine. If the stress cannot be reversed and becomes chronic, it can affect the release of hormones and cause low libido.

If you feel that life stress is affecting sexual desire, consider symptom management. From hiking to meditation or acupuncture, this could be anything. When you use specific strategies to prevent anxiety and stress from affecting your life, chronic stress will be reduced. Ultimately, this will contribute to stability. Discussing stress management with experts may help to apply the necessary coping techniques.

Another factor in low libido is relationship stress. Studies have shown that low sexual desire conflicts with the relationship between men and women. The lack of interest of one partner will affect the attention of another partner. Overcoming these difficulties is essential for many reasons, including sexual desire.

8. APPETITE CHANGES

Stress may cause a loss of appetite. Sometimes you may lose your appetite, and sometimes you may attack the refrigerator at night. Stress stimulates the brain to secrete hormones that activate the sympathetic nervous system. A stress hormone, called corticotrophin-releasing factor, can suppress appetite and reduce the body's natural hunger hormones. It is not uncommon for people with excessive stress to have elevated levels of this hormone in their bodies, resulting in a loss of appetite.

Not sure if stress will increase or decrease your appetite. It depends on the type or severity of the situation; you may eat more or less. In the final exam, you may want to eat a variety of junk food, but after breaking up with your boyfriend, you may have a complete loss of appetite. It is not entirely clear why this happens, but it may be related to stress hormones and their effects on hunger and satiety.

Some women feel sick when eating under pressure. This may result in a decreased appetite. Once individuals are convinced that this is how their bodies react when they eat under pressure, it may become a habit that further exacerbates this cycle.

Another effect of stress on food is a sense of control. Some women may start restricting and overeating because controlling food may help relieve anxiety. Stress can cause eating disorders, so it's important to keep mindfulness during this time.

9. MUSCLE TENSION

Muscle tension is often experienced under stress. This may cause short-term stiffness or stiffness for hours or even days until the stress is relieved or help is sought. The degree and severity may vary from person to person. Many women with stress have pain in the back, neck, shoulders, or chest. Some women may find that muscle tension is affecting their quality of life. It is important to seek medical attention to manage muscle tension.

10. RAPID HEART BEAT

Everyone feels stress in different ways. When the stress is too high, high blood pressure or heart often occurs. Because stress hormones are irritants, the brain releases hormones that cause the heart to beat. These hormones include epinephrine and cortisol. They enter your bloodstream, increase your heart rate, and may eventually lead to the heart.

Many factors trigger stress. The consequences of constant stress and internal tension cannot be understated. The psychological and physiological effects of stress influence each other and promote each other. This created a cycle that affected more and more people.

Key facts at a glance:

Chronic stress puts the body in a state of permanent activation, which leads to exhaustion.

People who are chronically stressed are at higher risk of heart disease or stroke.

Inner tension and concentration are the first psychological consequences of stress.

The body's response to stress

The body releases hormones adrenaline and cortisol under pressure. These can activate the body and prepare for battle or escape reactions. All parts of the body are affected.

Under stressful conditions, the bronchial tubes expand to absorb more oxygen. This makes breathing quick and shallow. Also, the heart beats faster and stronger, which increases blood pressure and narrows blood vessels. Muscles can also supply blood better and are tenser. Overall, the body is prepared to increase energy expenditure and release more sugar into the blood. On the other hand, digestion is delayed, and pain sensitivity is reduced. In this way, the whole body is ready to take action.

After the dangerous situation is over, hormone production decreases, and the body returns to calm. However, if you continue to apply pressure, you will not be able to recover fully. This means that you are always in this state of excitement. Over time, this can lead to exhaustion or other physical and psychological problems.

PHYSICAL CONSEQUENCES OF HIDDEN STRESS IN WOMEN

Without adequate recovery, stress can affect your overall health and thus permanently alter the body. Psychological stress should not be underestimated either.

Brain and ears

There is constant stress throughout the body. This has particularly lasting consequences in the brain. Under short-term stress, the performance of the brain will increase. But under long-term stress, it will overload in the long run. Therefore, the mass of the brain shrinks, and the branches of the brain decrease. This will also deteriorate memory performance. In the worst case, chronic stress can lead to a stroke.

The sensory organs also respond to stress. Ear pressure symptoms appear tinnitus and even sudden hearing loss. With tinnitus, the affected person can hear the tone without an external sound source. Depending on how you feel, this may have a significant impact on life. Hearing loss can cause unilateral hearing loss. It may be caused by ear circulation disorders, which may be related to stress. However, the theory has not been scientifically proven. In addition to stress, physical causes can also cause tinnitus or sudden hearing loss. In this case, you should always ask your doctor to check for these symptoms.

Cardiovascular System

Chronic stress can weaken the cardiovascular system. Researchers have found that people with long-term stress suffer from cardiovascular disease twice as often as people with stress.

Typical symptoms are:

Hypertension
Increased blood lipid levels
Increased sediment on ships
All these factors increase the risk of heart attack. The heart rhythm may also be disordered. Common feelings are:

Racing heart or stumbling
Dizziness
Chest pain

Upset stomach

The gastrointestinal tract also feels the effects of stress. As the number of stress hormones increases, the body produces more stomach acid. As a result, patients are more vulnerable to heartburn.

The risk of stomach ulcers is also higher. However, if the gastric mucosa is already inflamed, chronic stress can only cause ulcers. For example, an increase in stomach acid can cause this inflammation. Typical complaints that follow:

- stomach ache
- nausea
- Satiety
- Loss of appetite
- A further consequence of gastrointestinal pressure is chronic digestive problems, such as B. Constipation or diarrhea.

Diabetes

Stress is also considered a significant risk factor for diabetes, just like being overweight or not exercising. The hormone cortisol is released under stress. This increases blood sugar level and activates the body. The creature also releases messenger substances related to stress. These will reduce the effect of insulin, making it difficult to regulate blood sugar. Results: People who are under stress for a long time are more likely to develop diabetes.

You can identify diabetes by the following symptoms, including:

Thirst
Fatigue
Lose weight
Urge to urinate often

Poor wound healing
Weak immunity

When the body is in an alert state, the immune system will be strengthened in a short time. In this way, it can fight off infection faster. However, the stress hormone cortisol can permanently weaken the defense system of the immune system. Bacteria and viruses can attack organisms more quickly, and being rejected has little success. As a result, stressful people suffer more infectious diseases. Most of them have a cold or herpes. They also need a longer time to recover health.

Tense muscles

Because the body is always vigilant, the muscles are permanently tense. This tension is most pronounced in the head, shoulder, and back areas. The result is headache and back pain, and if they are not relaxed enough, they may become chronic stress. As a result, the body is tired and inefficient.

Increased skin disease

Women with neurodermatitis pay special attention to the effect of pressure on their skin. Permanent inflammation increases the typical skin inflammation of eczema and itching. To reduce stress, only scratching is usually helpful. However, this increases inflammation. Inhibiting itching increases internal tension. Without relieving stress, affected women will increasingly suffer from this disease.

Psoriasis and urticarial have similar symptoms. These will also increase due to permanent pressure.

PSYCHOLOGICAL CONSEQUENCES OF STRESS

In addition to the effects of stress on the body, patients also suffer from psychological problems. In the short term, the following complaints will appear:

- Inner tension and restlessness
- Difficult to concentrate
- tension
- irritability
- Dissatisfied

Fear and anger

Without sufficient recovery, permanent stress can lead to more serious mental illness. Overall well-being continues to decline. Anxiety and dissatisfaction are more common.

Panic attack

In a panic attack, the affected person is in a state of intense fear. This happens when there are too many stress factors at once. These attacks usually start without warning and last for a few minutes to half an hour.

Typical symptoms include:

Palpitation or Racing Heart

Sweating
Feeling dizzy, lightheaded or fainting
Hot flashes or showers
Shortness of breath, choking or shortness of breath
Feeling tight in the throat or chest
Nausea or abdominal pain

Physical illness may also trigger panic attacks. Therefore, please contact your doctor first. If the cause is psychological, psychological therapy will usually help.

Burnout

Burnout is describes as an exhausted emotional, mental, and physical state. Various personal or professional stress factors can trigger the disease. The symptoms of the disease may be physical or psychological.

Symptoms of physical burnout may include:

Fatigue, poor performance, poor concentration, forgetfulness, and irrecoverability.
Insomnia, heart pit at night
Neck tension, shoulder pain, external fingers wake up in the morning
Acidification, premature pain in the elbow (probably tennis elbow), wrist, knee or buttocks
Frequent lower back pain caused by standing work, sometimes sciatica will radiate to the legs
Tight stomach and hepatobiliary symptoms, frequent flatulence, severe fat intolerance, and chronic constipation

Insufficient defense capacity due to stress, susceptibility to infection, cold sores, delayed inflammation of frontal sinus inflammatory mucus and persistent headache caused by cough
Hoarseness of chronic vocal cords caused by mucus
Weather-sensitive circulatory system problems, cold hands, and feet
Side effects of many antibiotic treatments include immunodeficiency (destroying the intestinal flora, producing 70% of the non-specific defense system), abdominal cramps, diarrhea, and long-term intestinal mycosis (Candida albicans)

The psychological symptoms are:

Excited spirit, uneasy
Shutdown problems that make it hard to fall asleep
Depressed mood, depressed
Concentrate and forget
Increased demand for harmony
Con conscience within, worried about failure due to declining performance
Increased turmoil in the private sector

Only in the interaction between physical and mental aspects can you get to the bottom of the complications. Psychotherapy can also help those with the exhausted syndrome. Depending on the patient's condition, you can also use mood-enhancing drugs for treatment.

Burnout syndrome does not develop overnight. Instead, it is based on a one-year process in which burnout syndrome will gradually develop.

As a person seeking exhausted advice, you are at a crossroads of ten road signs. These lead to ten types of fatigue discovered by Dr. Mansman in his many years of work.

TEN TYPES OF FATIGUE

1. "Depressive weakness syndrome."

The causes of this fatigue are permanent psychological stress, sadness, anxiety and fear, and shocking experiences. Depression is a typical clinical manifestation.

How can it help? According to Dr. Wearer's exercise therapy, ultraviolet radiation, and homeopathy. If it is the cause of menopausal hormone disorders or liver disease, it must be treated accordingly.

2. "Overwork Syndrome."

Overwhelmed-this makes sense. But stress is not so easy! If we completely get rid of the pressure, we will shrink. Stress creates resilience and keeps us resilient at "normal doses." The heartbeat before the meeting is an example of positive pressure (also called Eu pressure). Anger, hatred, anger, jealousy, or jealousy is examples of negative pressure or low mood. When stress persists for a long time, and the body and mind cannot adapt, mental failure occurs. The resilience is much lower than normal, and the diseases no longer heal

themselves: they build nests and become chronic diseases.
Now permanent damage may occur.

How can it help? According to Dr. Wearer's exercise therapy,
manual muscle therapy, shiatsu massage, and permanent
shower. Plan a day, spending 15 minutes a day, plan the
relaxation phase, and stay active and social. Mediation and
yoga classes, various anti-stress techniques.

3. "Immune Deficiency Syndrome."

The law of stress and insanity does not only apply to the
entire body. You can observe each organ from this angle. This
fatigue may be due to weakened organs, psychological causes,
or intestinal immune system disorders, such as indirect
damage (malnutrition) caused by intestinal fungi or antibiotics.

How can it help? Control the symbiosis in the intestine, take
a fresh shower every day, do endurance exercise, take a sauna
once a week, eat fewer sweets. Immune-enhanced herbal
products (Echinacea) or bee products (bee pollen, royal jelly,
propolis) are suitable for short-term treatment.

4. "Circulatory muscle weakness syndrome."

Symptoms of this fatigue include getting up in the morning,
dizziness when standing, dizziness after bending down or
standing for a long time, headache, sensitive weather,
difficulty concentrating early in the morning, or difficult
hours studying in the first school.

How can it help? Ginseng, guarana, mate, enzymes, echinacea, bee pollen, royal jelly, propolis.

5. "Hormonal Disorder Syndrome."

Chronic fatigue may be a symptom of hypothyroidism. In the most harmless case, the cause is diet-related iodine deficiency. The low mood during menopause may indicate that peristaltic ovarian inflammation has not been detected, and there is a lack of female hormones. Very rare causes may be adrenal disease (Addison's disease) or pituitary gland (pituitary gland) disease, such as Cushing's syndrome.

How can it help? Only your therapist can determine the exact cause. According to the reasons, the following measures are recommended: black cohosh, St. John's wort, royal jelly, and sea fish twice a week, and iodine tablets containing iodine.

6. "Weak Metabolic Syndrome."

All organs involved in digestion help to obtain energy from food. The abnormal health of these organs can lead to a lack of energy (exhaustion). In particular, in this type of fatigue, the function of the liver, gallbladder, pancreas, or intestine is disturbed.

How can it help?

Liver disease: Milk thistle capsules, continuous homeopathy

For weak galls: gall tea, garlic, and artichoke preparations
For chronic constipation: herbal laxative tea, bran, alfalfa
tablets, and walking

7. "Malnutrition syndrome."

Despite the prosperity, malnutrition and typical fatigue
increased again. Fast food, over-fertilized agriculture, dishes
cooked in a microwave oven, or long-term insulation (meals
in the canteen) can all cause vitamins to cook. The elderly are
particularly affected because they only eat a small portion
anyway and therefore consume minimal vitamins overall.

How can it help? Nutritional recommendations, chewable
fruit and vegetable tablets, no smoking, moderate drinking.

8. "Poisoning and Allergy Syndrome"

The cause of this fatigue is the contamination of our immune
system with live poisons, such as contaminants in carpet glue
or wall coatings, wood preservative poisons, and side effects
of drugs or allergic reactions to certain foods. This leads to
weak defense and fatigue quickly.

How can it help?

In case of poisoning: remove it by homeopathic remedies, for
example, and remove poisons from living areas [Caution. d.
Editor: Panchakarma therapy is also very interesting here; it

can promote relaxation and excretion at the same time and can
help give life new vitality and enthusiasm when burning.
Allergies: calcium, homeopathy, symbiotic control,
immunostimulation methods

9. "Chronic Disease Syndrome."

Continual exposure to chronic diseases (such as diabetes,
anemia, arteriosclerosis, or other chronic intestines, lungs, or
heart disease) can be the cause of this fatigue.

Without a definitive diagnosis by a doctor, it is impossible to
recommend any treatment plan.

How can it help?

Diabetes: Silybum marianum, acupuncture treatment of eye
diseases, Ginkgo biloba promotes blood circulation
Iron Deficiency: Homeopathy

10. "Chronic Fatigue Syndrome (CFS)"

This diagnosis is a collective term. This includes fatigue states
that meet certain typical criteria but cannot be assigned to a
certain disease.
How can it help? Without a doctor's precise diagnosis, there is
no treatment recommendation here.

HIDDEN FEAR IN WOMEN

Those who are not afraid are not alive! Fear is a part of our lives and is essential to our development. Everyone is scared of other things: examinations, diseases, individual animals, loneliness, crowds, embarrassment, etc. Fear is a natural and useful protection mechanism: it enables us to react quickly in dangerous situations. After that, tensions usually subside as soon as they are established.

When fear lasts for an unusually long time, it will become a disease, affected people will not be able to control it, and the outside world will not be able to identify physical causes. Sometimes, patients do not even realize their fears because they only focus on physical symptoms. Therefore, anxiety disorder is hidden behind many mental and physical discomforts.

Anxiety triggers a physiologically similar stress response: the hypothalamus controls the formation of cortisol, which regulates the metabolism of fats, carbohydrates, and proteins. The adrenal glands produce more epinephrine and norepinephrine, thereby accelerating the body's energy supply within seconds: increased heart rate and blood pressure, which increases blood flow to the muscles, but the brain is virtually "turned off."

Anxiety women usually have elevated levels of adrenaline in their blood. The slightest situation is enough to trigger a fear reaction among them. The pulse rises, blood drains from the face, they tremble, and their knees become weak. Their

breathing becomes faster, but they feel unable to breathe.
Some women are afraid that they may even experience
stomach pain when vomiting or diarrhea. Other physical
symptoms of anxiety include wide pupils, sweating, urgency,
headache, dizziness, and fainting.

Affected women do not need to be aware of their fears, but
sometimes cause a lot of physical discomforts. Among other
things, they lead to:

- Digestive problems (flatulence, constipation, diarrhea)
- Sleep, eating, and inattention
- Heart problems caused by arrhythmia, maybe until a
  heart attack
- Difficulty breathing to asthma
- incontinence
- Depression
- Increased sensitivity to infection

The doctor's difficulty is to realize that fear is the cause of the
patient's physical discomfort. Even if the affected people
know their fears, they usually will not admit it publicly
(hidden "fear.") For some of the effects of fear, doctors can
prescribe medicine, and only psychological therapy can bring
the ultimate relief.

HIDDEN DEPRESSION

Depression is a serious mental illness. The patient felt very depressed, lost interest, exhausted, and lack of energy. The disease lasts for a long time and usually cannot improve on its own without treatment.
Depression often surrounds the affected people like a black curtain. With the right combination of psychotherapy and medicine, you can start again!

Depression is a serious mental illness and should be treated professionally. Unlike sadness and listlessness in life, depression does not disappear on its own after a while, nor does it improve by distracting or encouraging.

Depression is a persistent state of mind that affects thinking, feeling, and behavior. If the typical symptoms have been present for at least two weeks, the disease is diagnosed. The affected people usually feel depressed and feel empty. They also lose interest in hobbies or professions and no longer feel happy. Another symptom is lack of energy: the patient is weak and tired.

Patients with chronic pain usually become depressed. But there are also opposite cases: in 5-10% of all cases, pain indicates mental illness. If physical discomfort is so important that the doctor can hardly identify the psychological cause, it can be said to be larvae or hidden depression.
With severe depression, negative thoughts can become so intense that thoughts of suicide arise. The risk of suicide is

very high in some depressed people. About ten to fifteen
percent of patients with depression die from suicide

Women suffer from depression two times as often as men. A
possible explanation is that women are at higher risk due to
hormonal fluctuations (for example, before menstruation).

Profound hormonal changes can also cause pregnancy, which
can cause pregnancy depression in some women. The so-
called postpartum depression or postpartum depression also
encounters many women.

Low socioeconomic status is also a risk factor for depression-
there is more women in poverty than men.

Also, depression is less common in men. Some people avoid
showing weakness and seek help. But they also sometimes
have atypical symptoms, such as aggressiveness and excessive
behavior.

Those affected are unable to express their frustration. You
will always feel dull and often suffer from hot flashes or chills.
Their brain area, the so-called limbic system, constantly sends
out signals that make the muscles tense: the presence of
tension eventually leads to dysfunction and pain. Depending
on the affected area, patients will suffer from the following
typical symptoms:

- Gastrointestinal tract: nausea, vomiting, diarrhea,
  constipation, gas, loss of appetite

- Cardiac/circulatory system: beating heart, heart, anxiety, shortness of breath, dizziness, drowsiness
- Genitourinary system: sexual sensory dysfunction, dysfunction, menstrual bleeding
- Musculoskeletal system: lower back pain and neck pain
- Other symptoms may include:
- headache, tinnitus (tinnitus), visual impairment, itching (allergy), hair loss
- Attention and decreased attention
- Self-esteem and self-confidence decline
- Feeling worthless
- Negative and pessimistic thoughts
- sleep disorder

In most cases, drugs and psychotherapy are necessary to treat depression.
Doctors or psychotherapists can only discover hidden depressions by asking specific questions about the patient's mental state. And only the patient answered openly and honestly. It can be cured with psychotherapy and antidepressants.

When suffering from depression, too little serotonin and norepinephrine are produced in the brain. These messenger substances are responsible for signal transmission from one nerve cell to another. If they are gone, the person concerned will be frustrated. Within weeks to months, the messenger substance must be added to the body until it reaches a steady-state again. Physical discomfort disappears with depression.

12 SIGNS OF HIDDEN DEPRESSION

Depressed women are deeply saddened by only half of the truth because they can also smile magically, be punctual, or have a more philosophical meaning to life.

Contrary to popular belief, depression is not characterized by sadness, but by feelings of numbness and inner emptiness. So, what are the real signs of frustration? How do you identify hidden depression?

1. Show a smile-"smile depression."

Let's face it: women try to cover up the unpleasant feeling after a smirk. For example, maybe you are working, and colleagues should not be aware of your emotions, or you do not want to be a burden for friends. Smiles are always welcome; at least this is what many women believe.

However, smiles are healthy and beautiful only when there is the right emotion behind them, that is, joy. But when the smile masked the unpleasant sensation, it quickly turned into a mask, hiding the frustration. For example, Robin Williams smiled until he committed suicide.

The more you try to use a smile to disguise other feelings such as sadness, anger, fear, loneliness, or inferiority, the more frustration may appear behind a sympathetic smile. That takes the energy of a corset man or a huge woman; it may eventually lead people with depression to avoid contact with others.

The song "Don't worry, be happy"-"Don't be angry, be happy" may also be the guiding principle for people with depression. This is why this form of depression is also called "laugh depression" or "smile depression."

Laughter is the right way to deal with unpleasant emotions. Swiss psychoanalyst CG Jung wrote: "Humans will only get better if they talk about their dark side." So talking and crying can be a way to prevent or reduce depression.

2. Unreliable and fickle

Friends' phone: Warm questions about the joint meeting. There are many ideas about what you can do. What will happen? No! Because the affected women canceled at the last minute, the meeting was not held. Here, the pit will spread around the corner to prevent its undulation.

Unreliable, forgetful, and lazy...

... These may be personality traits that are not considered particularly "sexy." However, for depression, it has nothing to do with personality, but with the unreliable drive to indicate a reduction, which is a typical feature of depression. The reduced driving force is also attributed to the feeling of eternal life. This continued tension can also lead to excessive fatigue, which can cause the affected people to "unable to unite." Also, there may be problems with inattention, decreased performance, and numbness-from the outside, you think it is pure laziness or forgetfulness-but this lack of motivation is part of depression.

But this may also be very different, because women with depression may also look fickle. This expresses the inner uneasiness, which is physically "under the tide." On the one hand, the response to the environment is often a lack of understanding of internal motivation; on the other hand, the lack of knowledge of apparent comfort.

3. Sudden emotional outburst

The mood of women with depression changes every day, even during the day. Depressed women are also more sensitive to different living conditions, which can lead to intense mood swings and sudden emotional bursts. Men often respond with irritability, impulsivity, and aggressive attitudes, but women are also more likely to be irritable in depression than usual, and anger or sadness suddenly burst out. This strong mood swing may indicate masked depression. The inner tension seemed to disappear immediately. Women showed frustration, emotional despair, and helplessness. And the feeling of wanting to hide.

4. Unable to decide

"Should I or should not!?"-Women with depression often think about it. Somehow, the decision seems so tricky. Even if you choose with a few expected consequences. The hidden depression manifests as a feeling of being torn. Fear of making mistakes may make it impossible to make a decision.

Then began to meditate. Chewing the same thought again and again. They give you a headache. Thoughts are turning. But no results.

5. Hidden depression and eating behaviors

Anorexia is a typical depression. Taste is significantly reduced. This usually leads to severe weight loss. However, sometimes there are atypical changes in eating habits, namely food cravings (increased appetite, especially for carbohydrates, fats, high sugar, or high salt foods).

It can be said that depression lacks the sweetness of life-the the taste of life. Eating behavior attempts to balance the inner emptiness.

As a guideline for depression, the WHO (World Health Organization) stipulates a weight loss or weight gain of 5% compared to the previous month.

6. Fatigue and sleep behavior

Fatigue and substantial feelings like lead are typical signs of depression. "Getting up" requires a lot of effort, but women

With depression also often suffer from sleep disturbances.

Wake up late at night because you can't fall asleep or worry about missing something (challenging to fall asleep); suddenly wake up at night during sleep (difficult sleep), have nightmares or get up in the morning much earlier than usual, but the demand for sleep increases Or the feeling of having trouble getting up in the morning-changing sleep behavior may be a clear sign of depression. Conversely, depression also changes sleep behavior. This does not mean that depression can be suspected immediately after each sleep disorder. However, you should consult your doctor for restless sleep or restless sleep (feeling tired in the morning). Moreover, if possible physical causes can be ruled out.

Some antidepressants can induce sleep, and relaxation procedures (such as progressive muscle relaxation or self-training) can also help you sleep well.

7. Zero blog emotions, or "I don't care."

Not wanting to work may just mean that you have the wrong job or the wrong colleague. In principle, you can make some changes to this.

However, Zero Goat's mood is not easy to change, smile, or solve it by "getting up now." Anyone who tries to inspire someone's emotions will get "I don't care". Because the depression of the hand luggage is not so easy-it is always there, covered with the feeling of the affected person like a gray veil; the result is inner emptiness, "cold emotions" and rigidity.

8. Increase activities-sports, work, and forced discipline

As mentioned earlier, the lack of motivation is a typical manifestation of depression. However, for patients with recessive depression, especially they seem to suddenly increase their activities. Inner restlessness manifests itself physically, for example, through increased exercise (beyond health in time) or through extreme exercise (such as skydiving, no safe climbing, or bodybuilding (as over-optimized body worship)). It seems voluntary, and the increase in overtime work may also be a sign of disguise.

Women with depression not only often try to defeat black demons with their own strength at work, extreme sports and other activities, but also celebrate fixed rituals that should give those affected support in order to avoid depression in advance.
Since depression can also occur with eating disorders (such as anorexia or bulimia), as mentioned above, it should also be mentioned here that increased activity also affects eating behaviors. Scientists are currently studying the relationship between depression and a strong desire to eat as "healthy" as possible. There are also compulsive acts here.

9. Physical depression

Depression also manifests physically, for example:

Regular indigestion (irritable bowel, constipation, diarrhea, stomach cramps, heartburn, nausea, vomiting, flatulence)
Physical fatigue, fatigue, fatigue easily, fatigue
Feeling sick and unexplained
Hot flashes, chills, tremors
Chronic pain (usually a headache, migraine or back pain)
Muscle tone (neck and shoulder area, varicose veins)
Loss of appetite, craving, weight change
Sleep disorders
Feeling chest pressure, tightness, or "lump in the throat."
Dizziness, tinnitus, shortness of breath (usually combined with an anxiety disorder), shallow breathing, difficulty breathing, cardiovascular disease (rapid heartbeat, heartache, heartbreak syndrome)
Blinking eyes, blurred vision, allergy to light
Gritted teeth
Attention deficit, memory disorder, pseudo-dementia
Decreased libido (decreased libido), sexual dysfunction

. 10. Alcohol

One or two after-work beers or a glass of wine - You notice it!? These trivializations with "Chen" already illustrate the problem! Alcohol is and remains a pleasure poison, which should only be drunk in moderation, if at all.
Alcohol abuse begins small, with a glass of wine or a beer a day, and in the worst-case ends in delirium. Even if it is "just to fall asleep" or "to relax," women with hidden depression often try to treat themselves with alcohol. A dangerous game, because it often leads to addiction.

11. Philosophy about the meaning of life and death

Everyone is thinking about how life should develop. Especially when there are significant changes (such as separation or job changes), it is important to waste time thinking about how to set up routes in the future.

On the other hand, a woman who hides frustration not only thinks about the future but also has many philosophical thoughts about the meaning of life. Death was also discussed. But sometimes there are still thoughts about suicide. For women with depression, suicidal thoughts have increasingly become the center of the thinking world. For the environment, it is essential to wake up and listen when bleak prospects for the future appear in the topics discussed. Psychologists describe this phenomenon as "depressive realism," which loses its realistic view of itself and the environment.

12. "I'm fine" or "okay" attitude

Losing (due to separation, unemployment, or lack of health) and feeling sad, disappointed, and injured are natural and healthy. But this will usually be resolved a few weeks later. However, if the black hole persists for weeks or appears suicidal, you should take it seriously and seek support.

Women with depression mainly do this by: "I get along well. I'm in a bad mood now." Out of shame, fear of rejection, or sometimes just because they don't want to be a burden on anyone, they try to make their feelings trivial or hidden. This false reluctance will only unnecessarily prolong the suffering of those affected.

Depression can be cured. Most depression occurs in stages. Rapid treatment can significantly shorten the duration of the so-called depression period, which also reduces the risk of another type of depression.

In addition to psychotherapy, antidepressants can also be used. It should be discussed with the attending doctor. The tendency to return to depression persists, especially if depression has been diagnosed in the past, exhaustion or burnout.

Depression treatment

Statistics shows that one out of three people will feel depressed in their lives. Rapid treatment is very important because the affected people have suffered a lot. Also, treatment becomes more difficult, and the risk that the disease becomes chronic increases.

Depending on the severity of the disease, depression can usually be treated with psychotherapy, antidepressants, or a combination of both. The combination therapy is particularly suitable for chronic and recurrent depression. Even with severe depression, experts still recommend a combination of the two treatments.

Psychotherapy for depression

There are many psychotherapy services for people with depression. However, at present, health insurance companies only bear the costs of cognitive-behavioral therapy and so-called psychodynamic psychotherapy.

Psychotherapy

Psychotherapy requires a few months of patient patience and input. However, if you are involved, you can usually overcome depression for a long time and improve your overall psychological stability.

Cognitive behavior therapy

Through cognitive-behavioral therapy, patients look for ways to get rid of depression with the support of the therapist. Among other things, discover negative thoughts, patterns, and beliefs, check their correctness and replace them with more positive new ways of thinking when necessary.

Psychodynamic psychotherapy

Psychodynamic psychotherapy is based on the idea that depression is normally caused by loss and insulting experiences that cannot be handled properly. These should be dealt with during treatment. Psychodynamic psychotherapy includes classic psychoanalysis and psychotherapy based on deep psychology.

Other forms of psychotherapy for depression

Interpersonal therapy (IPT) is a short-term therapy developed specifically for the treatment of depression. It combines the treatment concepts of behavioral therapy and psychodynamic therapy. An important therapeutic goal is to learn the skills and strategies to deal with conflicts that lead to the development or maintenance of depression.

However, the cost of ITP has not been borne by the health insurance company. This also applies to other therapies of verscheidene, such as systemic therapy, home therapy, Gestalt therapy, or art therapy. However, in the context of hospitalization, they are often used as supportive therapy.

This also applies to complementary treatments such as psychological education, occupational therapy, family groups, learning relaxation techniques, and body and exercise-related therapies.

Depression: drug treatment

Antidepressants can successfully treat the symptoms of depression. The effect usually only takes a few weeks. Drugs are usually prescribed for intense depression or patients who oppose psychotherapy.

However, there is no guarantee that the drug will achieve the desired effect. Everyone reacts differently to active ingredients: some beneficial effects are great, others have little effect, or most importantly, patients experience side effects.

If the drug is stopped, there will be a risk of relapse-especially if it happens suddenly. Therefore, do not stop taking antidepressants yourself, but discuss the procedure with your doctor!

Selective serotonin reuptake inhibitors (SSRIs)

Selective serotonin reuptake inhibitors (SSRI) or serotonin-norepinephrine reuptake inhibitors (SNRI) are currently used to treat depression. They can increase the level of serotonin "happiness hormone" in the brain, and have the effect of enhancing mood. The side effects of the drug are significantly smaller than the old drugs. Typical side effects include nausea, restlessness, and sexual dysfunction.

Tricyclic antidepressants

Tricyclic antidepressants are one of the oldest drugs used to treat depression. However, they have strong side effects like dry mouth, tremor, fatigue, and constipation. Arrhythmia and rapid heart rhythm can also occur, especially in the elderly. Therefore, tricyclic antidepressants are almost prescribed only when the new drugs are ineffective.

Monoamine oxidase inhibitor

Monoamine oxidase inhibitors (MAO) have also long been used to treat depression. They have similar side effects as tricyclic antidepressants. Special attention should be paid to the use of tranylcypromine. This active ingredient needs a strict low tyramine diet. For example, tyramine is present in dairy products, wine, and sausages. If patients do not avoid tyramine-rich foods, serious side effects may occur, such as high blood pressure.

Electroconvulsive therapy

With the help of electroconvulsive therapy, depression can usually be treated in the event that medication and psychotherapy fail. Short "seizures" are triggered by short-term current pulses under anesthesia. At first, this idea may be frightening. In fact, patients do not understand the procedure, and the risk is very low.

Guard therapy

The patient needs to stay awake in the second half of the next day or all night for treatment. You cannot cure depression with this method, but it can temporarily relieve symptoms. For a long time, even for a short time, the patient will feel good again. This is not only a huge relief but also makes them hope they can really overcome the frustration.

Depression-help women to help themselves.

Recent studies have concluded that assistance provided without direct contact with the therapist will also help. Self-help instructions are an option. Those affected can read a lot of information themselves and only occasionally contact experts who support them. For example, this can help shorten the waiting time for treatment.

Internet-based therapy and application

Another option is to provide professional advice on the
Internet. Use special computer programs for treatment. There
are now so-called depression apps and catboats that make it
easier to deal with depression. They are based on the elements
of cognitive-behavioral therapy.

Exercise as an antidepressant

Get out of the house and get out of depression! For depression,
experts also recommend regular physical exercise. This can
significantly reduce depression symptoms in the short and
long term. Regular exercise is as effective as antidepressants.
This can be explained by reducing stress and possibly
changing messenger substances such as serotonin and
norepinephrine.

But the psychological impact of sports may have a more
significant impact: patients get rid of the vortex of lack of
motivation and retreat. They experience that they can do
something for their mental health. Self-esteem is strengthened,
and despair is suppressed. Those who practices sports in small
groups will also benefit from the feeling of community and
social contact, a mood that usually becomes less and less in
depression.

Inpatient or outpatient depression treatment?

Mild or moderate depression can usually be treated by
outpatient psychotherapy. In the case of severe depression,
hospitalization, especially in the clinic, is necessary.

Medications, a wide range of psychotherapy options, and intensive care in the clinic, can help patients recover their structured daily lives.

If the risk of suicide is high, depressed people can also be admitted to the clinic against their will.

Physical illness and depression

Some physical illnesses can also exacerbate depression. Brain diseases and hormonal diseases, such as hyperthyroidism or hypothyroidism, especially affect the emotional world. For example, in Cushing's syndrome, the adrenal cortex releases excessive amounts of cortisol. The result is usually a depression period.

Severe and chronic diseases are also a permanent psychological burden. For example, people with cancer, severe cardiovascular disease, and diabetes often suffer from depression. Drugs used for treatment or physiological processes related to the disease may also increase the risk of depression.

On the contrary, depression may have an adverse effect on the progress of such diseases, and in some cases, even promote their development. Because of this combination of physical and mental illness, it is always important to treat mental and physical pain equally.

Depression and somatoform disorders

Depression also tends to be the so-called somatoform disorder. These are chronic diseases, and no natural cause can be found. Most importantly, this includes, for example, pain in the back, stomach, or joints. But indigestion, heart problems, or breathing problems may also be somatic.

Other mental illnesses

Women with depression often suffer from other mental illnesses. It is also important to identify the two diseases and treat them accordingly. These include

- anxiety
- Obsessive-compulsive disorder
- alcoholism
- Personality disorder
- Eating disorders

Winter depression: caused by lack of light

Some people get depressed only during the dark season-but they get depressed every year. Winter depression is a seasonal affective disorder (SAD). Symptoms such as listlessness, loss of interest, and depression are basically the same as those of classic depression, but they are usually mild. Strong sleep needs and cravings for sweets are also typical of further depression. This is why people with depression in winter usually gain weight in winter.

It is believed that the cause of this disease is the lack of sunlight, and some people are particularly sensitive to it. In the dark, the body releases large amounts of the sleep hormone melatonin. This hormone not only makes you tired but also makes you feel depressed.

The most important therapy for preventing and treating winter depression is light therapy. It reduces the period of depression, especially in winter depression. To this end, the patient should sit in front of a device that emits strong artificial sunlight, with 30 to 60 minutes of the sunrise every day for two weeks, until before sunrise and after sunset. If this is not enough, then additional medications and psychotherapy can also help.

Medicines and drugs

Taking certain medications can also affect your mood. These include cardiovascular drugs such as beta-blockers, but also cortisone and related substances, hormonal contraceptives, and some neurological drugs such as anti-epileptics and Parkinson's drugs.
Drugs such as alcohol, cannabis, and other substances that affect the psyche can also promote the onset of depression.

Bipolar disorder

Once the manic and depressive phases occur together, the bipolar disorder occurs. This is also one of the emotional disorders, but strictly speaking, this is not depression. The affected person then swings between two emotional extremes: frustration and lack of motivation on the one hand, and extreme euphoria, overconfidence, and exaggerated activism

on the other. Bipolar disorder is usually more difficult to treat
than classic depression.

HIDDEN ILLNESS

When we find ourselves overwhelmed or uncomfortable,
many of us may try to hide it. Whether we don't want to worry
about the people around us or want to spend a stressful week
at work, anyone can cover up snuff, cough, or pain from time
to time.

However, women are more likely to conceal their condition
often, thereby increasing health risks. Traditionally, women
are seen as caregivers in the family, and this preconceived
notion makes them more likely to try "difficult coping"
instead of seeking care. Whether it's working long shifts while
catching a cold, or concealing flu symptoms and pretending to
be okay, many women try to work through infections.

When women hide disease, they may make themselves more
likely to suffer from a serious illness in the future. Hidden
symptoms can make it harder to tell whether a cough is cold
or severe bronchitis. This makes it essential not only for
women to take care of themselves properly but for friends and
family to encourage women to get the rest they need.

What stress affects

Although it is easy to see that hidden disease symptoms may
be harmful to your health, it may be more difficult to
distinguish why stress is such an influencing factor. After all,
everyone sometimes feels pressure. A small amount of stress

may be a natural motivation for people to complete their work. However, not all stress is normal. When someone feels overwhelmed, it is essential to have a channel or person to negotiate with.

Similar to the trend of hiding symptoms of common diseases, many women also tend to hide severe stress. When women feel overwhelmed or particularly stressed about something, they may try everything well. This can be harmful to both mental health and physical health, as unresolved stress can cause an increase in blood pressure and increase the risk of serious diseases such as heart disease or stroke.

How to encourage wellness

When women in the family feel overwhelmed, please give support: Show compassion and remind you of women in your life that they have no burden on others, and their feelings are important. This will help them open up without having to worry about getting along with their loved ones.

If the women in your life seem to be sick, please express your concern to them: Tell them that you want to make sure they are okay and willing to provide help to take care of them. The spouse can take the initiative to take on the duties of parents and the chores at home. In contrast, the children can take action to take on extra trivial tasks so that the most important women in life have the opportunity to rest and recover.

When a woman is sick or feels too stressed, the woman should express her needs more clearly: For some people, this may be challenging, but it is essential to remember that maintaining health is part of maintaining the health of the entire family. Women should not be afraid of screaming when they need to rest. When they feel overwhelmed, they should seek help from relatives.

Take some time for self-care: This is not limited to taking medicine or sleeping after a cold. It should be included in your weekly routine. Self-care is a small way for women to take care of their bodies and stress regularly. Meditation time can be as short as 15 minutes or as broad as a spa day at home, but no matter which self-care technique you try; personal relaxation must be a top priority.

Find a healthy store: To relieve stress, find a healthy way out when you are frustrated or overwhelmed. This may be like participating in sports or physical activities. It can be engaged in crafts. Any method that can help someone relieve stress in a safe environment is an excellent way to solve the overwhelming stress.

Actively change lives: If frequent stress is a problem for you, then it may be time to change your schedule. If women often feel overwhelmed, they should consider their daily work and discuss with their loved ones how to make positive changes. It may shift housework or cut certain stressful activities. Women can change things in their lives that can be controlled to help improve stress levels.

Since women not only have to express their stress and get the TLC they need when they are sick, this is essential, so everyone in the family can do something to help you. Friends, family members, and women themselves can try the following methods to reduce the burden of internal stress and disease:

Taking women and their welfare as the top priority at home can significantly help relieve stress and take proper care of illness. When all the family knows how to do it, they can work together to ensure that mothers, grandmothers, aunts, sisters, and even friends can take care of themselves.

THE HIDDEN ILLNESS OF POSTPARTUM DEPRESSION

Pregnancy and childbirth are a powerful and demanding experience that causes significant structural, neurological, hormonal, and emotional changes in the mother's body. These changes usually cause imbalances and disharmony in the body, make new mothers vulnerable, and may weaken thoughts and feelings.

Having a baby usually brings exciting and joyful times, but postpartum psychosis can prevent mothers from having such joy. The voice of new mothers suffering from postpartum depression is usually silent. In today's social media, the stress faced by new mothers and the stress of shame due to lack of contact or lack of full happiness in childbirth will keep silent.

Defining postpartum depression

The three most common postpartum diseases are postpartum depression or "infant depression" (considered normal postpartum adjustment), postpartum depression (PPD), and postpartum psychosis. Postpartum depression is the most common emotional disorder affecting women after childbirth. It affects up to a quarter of women in North America and is often confused with "depression." The symptoms of postpartum depression are more intense and influential than "infant depression." They will last longer, which hinders the mother's health and ability to take care of herself and her baby. This severe emotional disorder is a complex disease with extensive symptoms. The presentation can start at any time after delivery, and according to most researchers, it can last up to a year.

Symptoms of postpartum depression include, but are not limited to: negative feelings, fatigue, fragility, tearing, irritability, internal, discomfort, depression, self-awareness, despair, anxiety (such as unexplained concerns about your baby's health), hostility towards yourself The child or the joy of the mother feels trapped in responsibility, exhaustion, lack of motivation, systemic symptoms (including rapid heartbeat, sweating, nausea, dizziness, panic), loss of appetite, stomach pain and indigestion.

In some cases, people find that depression and worsening symptoms will escalate to postpartum psychosis, which is a very serious mental illness manifested as the idea that mothers are hurting themselves or babies. In these cases, immediate medical attention is necessary.

Things to consider

The diagnosis of postpartum depression can be difficult, and treatment is usually delayed. Social stigma on mental illness, confusion in diagnosis and feelings of shame, sense of inner and embarrassment often cause mothers to reduce symptoms, delay treatment, and remain silent.

After this extreme physical and emotional transition and strong hormonal, psychological, and biological changes, many factors should be considered. These considerations include biological mechanisms (such as changes in biochemical and hormonal factors), pathological mechanisms of neurotransmitter or receptor levels, hormonal disorders and thyroid dysfunction, and the bidirectional relationship between the immune system and the hypothalamic-pituitary-adrenal axis Association (HPA) / Hypothalamic-pituitary-gonadal axis (HPG), micro nutrition, biomechanical considerations and dislocations, and socioeconomic factors in labor and postpartum labor.

Traditional treatment options for postpartum depression may include: antidepressants, cognitive behavioral therapy, interpersonal relationship therapy, psychodynamic therapy, and support counseling. In some cases, successful alternatives have been found to include: psychoneuroimmunology to reduce maternal stress and inflammation, as well as herbal supplements, exercise and hands-on therapies, such as osteopathy.

Osteopathic treatment of postpartum depression

Each postpartum clinical manifestation is unique and requires multiple treatments to re-establish overall body health and vitality.

Osteopathic therapy can include: spinal and pelvic mobilization, visceral manipulation, treatment involving the cranial-unit of the brain and spinal cord, and psycho-neuroendocrine immune unit.

How does bone disease help postpartum depression patients:

• Synchronous hormone
• Limit sleep disorders
• Normalization of neuroendocrinology (including thalamus, hypothalamus, pituitary, heart, thymus, adrenal gland, thyroid, ovary)
• Restore the dislocation of the musculoskeletal system and reduce pain (including coccyx, buttocks, pelvis, bones, spine, skull, ribs, lower limbs)

• Normalize the location, activity, and vitality of internal organs and organs (including the uterus, intestinal system, bladder, liver, and kidneys)
• Improve hormones, digestion, nutrient absorption, eliminate toxins and enhance immunity
• Detox
• Improve lymphatic drainage, circulation, distribution of nutrients and hormones
• Improve spinal cord, nervous system and brain activity
• Normalize emotions and improve emotions/motivation through the limbic system
• Stable nervous system
• Adjust chest and abdominal pressure

EATING DISORDER IN WOMEN

Secrets can prevent us from sharing too many things, but some secrets may cause us great harm. Eating disorders are a severe health problem, and affected women will do their utmost to keep them away from everyone. They affect all races and ethnicities with the highest mortality rate of all mental illnesses.

Women with eating disorders will tell you that they are unwilling to share their problems with family members, friends, or medical professionals.

Hide behind food

We are happy to make a good meal for you, but don't eat it yourself. Some of us are good at playing hide-and-seek games.

Don't touch the food on our plates, hide the green beans in a napkin, and move the food around, so it seems that we have eaten more. A small portion is our bread and butter, and we will have some snacks before the big meal!

How did it start?

Eating disorders may start over some time or may develop into eating disorders within a few months after life events such as school dances or beach trips. Eating disorders are so common that one out of every 100 American students fights against it. Among boys and girls, anorexia is more common than boys and men. This disease has nothing to do with food, but with self-worth.

Risky

Womenshealth.gov outlines the following risks:

- Girls between the ages of 13 - 19 and young women in their 20s are the most vulnerable.
- Eating disorders are also increasing among older women. In one study, 13% of American women over the age of 50 showed signs of eating disorders
- warning sign
- Eating habits (only eat certain foods)
- Skip meal
- No food touch
- Check the mirror for visible defects
- Extreme mood swings

- Sleep problems

How does it affect women?

If you are anorexia, your body cannot get the energy it needs from food, so it will slow down and stop working overtime. It can affect your body in the following ways:

- Heart problems, low blood pressure, slow heart rhythm
- Thinning of bones (decreased bone mass or osteoporosis)
- Kidney stones, kidney failure
- Lack of time may cause pregnancy problems
- Miscarriage during pregnancy, cesarean section, and a higher risk of low birth weight
- Anemia (when your red blood cells cannot deliver enough oxygen to the body) and other blood problems.

Fight against the disease!

Make a treatment plan that you and your doctor designed together. Take all treatment courses and follow the diet plan. Practice smart eating habits with fruits and vegetables. Don't try to hide your body under inappropriate clothes. Choose styles and clothing that make you feel good. Recovery is a difficult task, but with the support, you can become healthier and more energetic. Always remember that you are strong, confident, and your beauty comes from within.

CONCLUSION

The whole body feels stressed. Therefore, a permanent load may cause serious illness, such as: suffering from diabetes, gastric ulcer, or arrhythmia. Existing diseases may worsen.

Psychological influence should not be underestimated either. Dissatisfaction, nervousness, or fear can lead to more serious mental illness. Therefore, you should counteract daily stress and take a break from time to time.